Dr. Oleksandr Gerasymovych

Dangerous

Vaping

Abbreviations

AFOP - acute fibrinous and organizing pneumonia

ARDS - acute respiratory distress syndrome

BAL - bronchoalveolar lavage

BBB - Blood-Brain Barrier

CBD - cannabidiol

CDC - Centers for Disease Control and Prevention

COVID-19 - Coronavirus disease 2019

DNA - Deoxyribonucleic acid

EC - electronic cigarette

ECDC - European Center for Disease Control and Prevention

ECMO - Extracorporeal membrane oxygenation

EIS - Epidemic Intelligence Service

ELISA - enzyme-linked immunosorbent assay

EMT - Epithelial-mesenchymal transition

ENDS - electronic nicotine delivery systems

EVALI - e-cigarette or vaping use-associated lung injury

FDA - U.S. Food and Drug Administration

IARC - International Agency for Research on Cancer

IRF - Integrated Research Facility

NHBE - normal human bronchial epithelial cells

NIAID - National Institute of Allergy and Infectious Diseases

NIOSH - National Institute for Occupational Safety and Health

PAHs - polycyclic aromatic hydrocarbons

PEEP - positive end-expiratory pressure

PG - propylene glycol (propane-1,2-diol)

PHEIC - Public health emergency of international concern

PHIL - Public Health Image Library

THC - tetrahydrocannabinol

VEA - vitamin E acetate

VG - vegetable glycerine (propane-1,2,3-triol)

VOCs - volatile organic compounds

WHO - World Health Organization

ZEB - zinc finger E-box binding homeobox

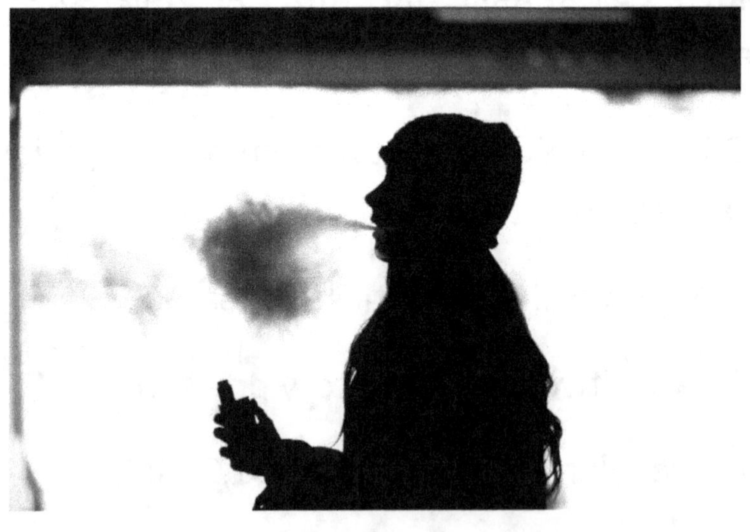

Index

About the author

Internal medicine doctor, graduated from Dnipro State Medical Academy in 2016, Ukraine. In 2018 I completed specialization in the city of Dnipro (in Internal Medicine). In 2012-2013 – internship in Italy (at the orthopedics and Internal medicine departments in Fabriano. On July 2021 - successful validation of the Ukrainian diploma at the University of Perugia in Italy. Author of the books "Coronavirus and arterial hypertension", "Prevention of coronavirus infection"; co-author of the books "Coronavirus and pregnancy", "Country 38 or Ukrainian anomaly", etc. In 2020, I received WHO certificates "Clinical management of SARI", "Prevention and control of novel coronavirus (COVID-19) infection". In November 2020, I attended a workshop on COVID-19 in Italy: "Do we share? Coronavirus, not just a clinical challenge" with the participation of microbiologists, an infectious disease specialist, an epidemiologist, internists, an anesthetist and an economist. In November-December 2020 - volunteering at the Department of Hygiene and Prevention of the Municipality of Perugia ("Contact tracing COVID-19" project) during the COVID-19 pandemic in the Umbria region. In May 2021 - participation in the seminar "Use of COVID-19 Vaccines: Explaining Rare Thrombosis with the AstraZeneca Vaccine" in Italy. I have participated in more than 30 conferences, including: XXIV Ukrainian Congress of Heart Surgeons, VI Scientific Session of the State Institution "Institute of Gastroenterology", Ukrainian Symposium "Pain Control", etc.

Other books of the author:

MonkeyPox (MPOX): How to Treat and How to Prevent, 2024 (amazon.com/dp/B0DG4C5TNX).

How to Treat Warts at Home, 2024 (amazon.com/dp/B0DGFCCSXT)

Orthonairoviruses and Wetland virus (WELV),2024 (amazon.com/dp/B0DGVH9W6Z)

Vaccines: Myths and Truths, 2024 (Ukrainian edition).

COVID-19 from A to Z, 2023 (amazon.it/dp/B0C2SH6KZV)

What experts say about my book "COVID-19 from A to Z":

"I was amazed by the "breadth" of the work, it is a truly remarkable review"

Roberto Burioni, Professor of Virology and Microbiology, Vita-Salute San Raffaele University, Milan.

"It seems to me to be a complete and well-documented text with a copious bibliography. I will suggest it to the students"

Prof. Fabrizio Pregliasco, Health Director of the IRCCS Galeazzi Hospital – Sant'Ambrogio, Full Professor of General and Applied Hygiene in the Section of Virology of the Department of Biomedical Sciences for Health of the University of Milan.

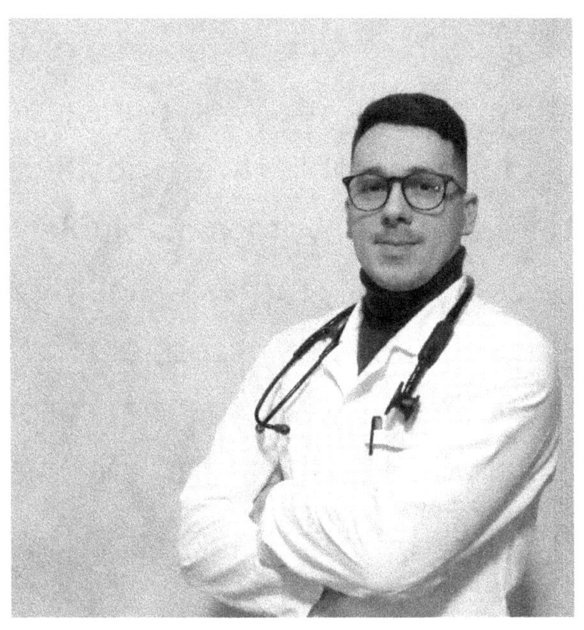

Introduction

Vaping is the process of inhaling and exhaling an aerosol produced by an e-cigarette, vape pen, or personal aerosolizer. When the device contains nicotine, the Food and Drug Administration (FDA) lists the product as an electronic nicotine delivery system or ENDS device.

Vaping or e-cigarettes involve high-temperature heating of a liquid to generate an aerosol vapor that can deliver substances, such as nicotine or tetrahydrocannabinol (THC), to the lungs. Generally, these liquids contain flavoring agents, diluents, nicotine, THC, nicotine and THC, or less typically, neither nicotine nor THC; the ingredients can vary greatly in chemical composition, especially between manufacturers or homemade mixtures. [82]

The most recent tobacco product that the general population is using more and more are electronic (e) cigarettes. [11-14] Even said, there is still a lack of knowledge on the impacts of vaping, or using e-cigarettes, and long-term usage of these devices is probably going to have detrimental effects on one's health. Over the past ten years, a range of e-cigarettes have been sold to the general population in the absence of regulatory action. The term "e-cigarette" or "vaping use-associated lung injury," or "EVALI," refers to a recently identified condition that is at the center of ongoing study and is an epidemic outbreak that has drawn attention to vaping devices from physicians and researchers. While vitamin E acetate (VEA), which is added to some vaping products, has been related to EVALI, aerosols produced by e-cigarettes (also known as electronic nicotine delivery systems, or ENDS) have the potential to cause numerous pulmonary toxicities, both acute and chronic.

Prior to EVALI, vaping had been associated with a wide variety of pulmonary presentations including lipoid pneumonia, acute respiratory distress syndrome, and diffuse alveolar hemorrhage. E-cigarette use can be profoundly hazardous. Exposure to EC aerosol can be even fatally harmful.

Prevalence of Vaping

Despite the high levels of nicotine and other additives in e-cigarettes, these devices have gained huge popularity among the general population, particularly among young adults, with an estimated 35 million users worldwide [86]. The United States (US) is by far the largest market for the consumption and utilization of e-cigarettes [87]. In fact, an estimated 8.1 million adults were using e-cigarettes in 2018 [88]. Alarmingly, the use of e-cigarettes among middle-and high-school students has seen a sharp increase since 2014 [89]. Funding for marketing campaigns on e-cigarettes also increased from $6.4 million spent in 2011, to $115.3 million in 2014 [90, 91], suggesting that as with traditional cigarettes, marketing strategies for e-cigarettes was predominately targeted toward adolescents. During 2014, e-cigarette advertisements reached approximately 18.3 million adolescents in the US [92]. Adolescents exposed to advertisements via the internet, in grocery stores, in print, and on TV were 1.52 times more susceptible to use e-cigarettes for the first time, and 2.22 times more likely to repeat use, if they were current users [93]. Vaping among middle-and high-school students has seen an exponential increase between 2017 and 2019, leading to the highest number of 5 million users in the year 2019 [94, 95].

E-cigarettes of today were created in 2003 and made their way onto the global scene in 2007 [11-14]. From the first-generation "cig-a-like," which was made to resemble a traditional tobacco cigarette, to the second-generation vape pens, the third-generation box mods, and the fourth-generation pod-based devices, which are currently quite popular, they have developed quickly [15, 16]. The hardware of these ENDS devices has rapidly evolved, but four essential parts have stayed the same: a mouthpiece [17], a power source (often a lithium rechargeable battery), an atomizer (heating element), and a liquid reservoir (also known as a tank, cartridge, or pod) to hold the e-liquid. However, each device is different in terms of temperature, power, metals, polymers, and other elements. Certain elements have been proven to be significant contributors to the generation of toxins. For example, applying high temperatures or wattages can produce high levels of formaldehyde, and wick length and coil design combinations can produce carbonyls. [18] Aerosols from e-cigarettes and e-liquids have also been shown to include toxic metals and other elements, which may be a result of the materials used to manufacture the devices. [19-21, 22-27]

Effects of Vaping on the body

There is conclusive evidence linking e-cigarette use with poisoning, immediate inhalation toxicity (including seizures), and e-cigarette or vaping product use-associated lung injury (EVALI; largely but not exclusively for e-liquids containing tetrahydrocannabinol and vitamin E acetate), as well as for malfunctioning devices causing injuries and burns. [104]

Adverse effects of electronic cigarettes on human health [1]:

- Eyes:

• Blurry vision

• Irritation;

 - Brain:

• Addiction

• Mood disorders

• Impulsiveness

• Hormonal imbalance;

• Seizures [97, 98]

• Syncope and tremors

• disrupts the integrity of the BBB [97, 98]

• increased risk of developing a stroke; [97, 98]

- Heart:

• Increased heart rate

- Hypertension

- Chest pain

- Arrhythmia

- Platelet activation and aggregation;

- Arterial stiffness [99]

- Angiogenesis and dyslipidemia; [100]

- Mouth:

- Gingivitis

- Periodontitis

- Microbiome imbalance;

- Para-tracheal edema, uvulitis, tonsilloliths, tonsillitis, and laryngitis; [98]

- Lungs and airway:

- Irritation

- Dry cough

- Increased airway resistance

• Increased inflammation and injury;

- Liver:

• Accumulation of fat;

- Stomach: Vomiting, nausea, acid reflux, abdominal pain;

- Kidneys: Reduced renal function.

Electronic Cigarette-Associated Pulmonary Syndromes[10]:

- Inhalation injury
- Exogenous lipoid pneumonia
- Hypersensitivity pneumonitis
- Acute eosinophilic pneumonia
- Diffuse alveolar hemorrhage
- Pneumothorax/pneumomediastinum
- Acute respiratory distress syndrome
- Respiratory bronchiolitis-interstitial lung disease
- Bronchiolitis obliterans
- Acute fibrinous pneumonitis
- Organizing pneumonia

- Granulomatous pneumonitis.

Mechanistic overview of the adverse effects of electronic cigarettes on the lung. As a primary organ, the lung is damaged and impaired by electronic cigarette use:

- overall effects on the lung: increased cytokines and chemokines, increased infiltration of inflammatory cells, increased activity of inflammatory cells, increased ROS and DNA damage (gammaH2AX), altered proteomics and transcriptomic profiles, altered cellular metabolism.
- effects on airway physiology: hyperreactivity, increased airway resistance, mucus hypersecretion, impaired ciliary beating, epithelial cell sloughing;
- effects on host defense: disrupted epithelial layer integrity, reduced macrophage phagocytosis, reduced bacterial clearance, reduced antiviral immunity. [1]

A wide range of lung diseases linked to vaping had been documented prior to 2019, including lipoid pneumonia, organizing pneumonia, diffuse alveolar damage and acute respiratory distress syndrome (ARDS), diffuse alveolar hemorrhage, hypersensitivity pneumonitis, peribronchiolar granulomatous pneumonitis, and the uncommon giant-cell interstitial pneumonitis. [38-42] The recent EVALI outbreak was distinct in that pathologic findings were consistent with a single common etiology, despite the possibility of a variety of pathologic presentations of respiratory injury brought on by inhaling aerosol from e-cigarettes. The majority of individuals with EVALI diagnoses (83%), reported using THC or CBD products manufactured with other terpene oils; the remaining 17% reported using solely vaping products that contain nicotine and are not frequently combined with terpenes, such as VEA. Blount and colleagues [43] discovered VEA in the bronchoalveolar lavage (BAL) fluid of 48 out of 51 EVALI patients in a convenience sampling, according to a research published in the New England Journal of Medicine. A few patients also had limonene and coconut oil detected. In 94% of this cohort, THC or its metabolites were detected in the BAL. VEA was discovered in 20 of the 20 bulk samples that law enforcement confiscated in 2019 but not in any of the 10 samples that they seized in 2018.

Lipid-laden alveolar macrophages, which usually accompany vacuolization and vacuolated pneumocytes, are common histopathologic characteristics in EVALI. [35, 43] Experiments conducted on animals have yielded preliminary data regarding the potential for acute lung harm caused solely by VEA exposure. [44] Numerous lipid-laden alveolar macrophages were seen in cells isolated from the BAL fluid of mice exposed to VEA; this finding is in line with clinical observations in patients with EVALI. [35, 43] Twenty-one of the suspected twenty-three cases in an autopsy series fit the EVALI criteria and exhibited histological evidence of acute to subacute lung injury, including organized pneumonia or diffuse alveolar damage. [45] Eight men, aged 19–61, who had respiratory symptoms after using e-cigarettes had transbronchial and surgical lung biopsies that revealed acute lung injury, including organized pneumonia and/or diffuse alveolar damage. [46] This is the predominant pattern in the acute process we call EVALI. Additional common features seen in the lung biopsies were fibroblast plugs, hyaline membranes, fibrinous exudates, type 2 pneumocyte hyperplasia, and interstitial organization. Some cases featured a sparse interstitial chronic inflammatory infiltrate. Although macrophages were present within the airspaces in all cases, this feature was not prominent, and findings typical of exogenous lipoid pneumonia were not present. [46]

It is yet unclear if youth vaping or cigarette smoking increases their risk of contracting COVID-19. In order to respond to this query, Gaiha et al. surveyed 4,351 teenagers and young adults (n = 13–24) nationwide via an online poll in May 2020. The study employed multivariable logistic regression analysis to investigate the associations among various variables, such as e-cigarette use exclusively, dual use (e-cigarettes and cigarettes), obesity, sociodemographic characteristics, and adherence to shelter-in-place protocols, and COVID-19-related symptoms, testing, and diagnosis. Five times more people were diagnosed with COVID-19 if they had never used e-cigarettes alone, seven times more if they had ever used dual cigarettes, and seven times more if they had used dual cigarettes for the previous 30 days. This study revealed that while COVID-19 is less common in youth, use of e-cigarettes only or the dual use of e-cigarettes and cigarettes increases the risk of COVID-19 in this demographic.

Vaping devices have potential impact on lung carcinogenesis. [81, 85, 96, 101, 102, 103] Association for the Study of Lung Cancer, in November of 2019, has issued a policy statement on e-cigarettes and vaping (https://www.iaslc.org/About-IASLC/News-Detail/iaslc-policy-statement---electronic-cigarettes).

Exposure to e-liquid also altered the expression of EMT markers [103]. Specifically, in A549 and H1650 cells exposed to e-liquid, expression of mesenchymal markers such as vimentin, fibronectin, zinc finger E-box binding homeobox (ZEB)1, and ZEB2 were induced [103].

Findings confirmed the association of e-cigarette use with cancer progression by inducing EMT transition and impairing DNA repair mechanisms. [85]

Some studies highlight the long-term neuroinflammatory consequences of developmental e-cigarette exposure. There was also a non-significant reduction in pup numbers and a decrease in fertility of male offspring, corroborating evidence from other studies that e-cigarette aerosol exposure causes a variety of potentially long-term detrimental health effects.

Kaisar, et al. (2017) found evidence of integrity impairment of the blood-brain barrier in mice acutely exposed to ENDS aerosol, which could further harm the functioning of the cerebral vasculature. [9]

Additive substances devoid of nicotine may induce cellular toxicity, which can lead to lung injury. For example, in well-differentiated primary normal human bronchial epithelial (NHBE) cells, it has been demonstrated that the flavoring compounds diacetyl and 2,3-pentanediol alone can disrupt transcriptome alterations associated with ciliogenesis and cytoskeletal structure. [51] Numerous cases of acute lung diseases, such as hypersensitivity pneumonitis, respiratory bronchiolitis-associated interstitial lung disease, and acute eosinophilic pneumonia, are found in the literature that are brought on by vaping nicotine-containing ENDS. [38, 45, 46]

As with cigarette smoking, the inhalation of chemicals contained within ENDS aerosols can elicit inflammatory responses in the lungs. Vaping has thus far been associated with asthma, [52-55] bronchiolitis, [45, 46] and alteration of airway defenses. [51] In the study including the Population Assessment of Tobacco and Health (PATH) study Wave 4 data on 33,606 US adult participants who indicated ever using e-cigarettes, the risk of wheezing and other respiratory symptoms was greater in ENDS users as compared to nonusers and lower compared to smokers. [56]

Inhalation of e-cigarette aerosol with nicotine caused altered transcriptomes of small airway epithelial cells and alveolar macrophages among all subjects and elevated plasma microparticle levels, providing in vivo human data demonstrating that acute inhalation of e-cigarette aerosols dysregulates normal human lung homeostasis in a limited cohort of healthy naïve individuals. [57]

Human exposure studies have also generally shown increased sympathetic nerve activity, platelet hemostasis processes, reactive oxygen species (ROS) generation, and endothelial dysfunction.

Adverse cardiac effects were also noted in a study of healthy, nonsmoking, and nonvaping adults who were exposed to secondhand vaping emissions. [33] These results were the first evidence of short-term, secondhand e-cigarette vapor-induced cardiac autonomic effects in healthy nonsmokers.

Although there are currently no human studies examining the effects of maternal ENDS use on birth or development outcomes, the main toxicants these devices emit raise serious public health concerns. [58] Despite having high levels of progesterone, a signal of pregnancy, the e-cigarette-exposed animals at day 5 showed almost no implantation sites, suggesting that the early pregnancy exposure of these female mice to e-cigarettes greatly impeded embryo implantation. [59] The effects of nicotine on the fetus are widely known; it is a major substance of concern in ENDS, but it is by no means the only one. [60-63] For this reason, the fetus may be seriously endangered by aerosols from both first- and second-hand e-cigarettes.

Nicotine use during pregnancy can have adverse health outcomes on the offspring's immune system, neural development, lung function, and cardiac function (England, et al., 2017).

Toxicant exposure from ENDS products may result in greater harm in adolescents than in adults (Wild & Kleinjans, 2003). Rubinstein, Delucchi, Benowitz, and Ramo (2018) indicated that while adolescent exposure to toxic volatile organic compounds (VOCs) was decreased in e-cigarette-only users versus dual users of e-cigarettes and traditional cigarettes, adolescent e-cigarette-only users still had levels of five different VOC toxicants detected in their urine in quantities up to three times greater than in matched controls. In addition to EVALI, multiple adverse health outcomes have also been associated with ENDS use, including bronchitic symptoms (chronic cough, phlegm, and bronchitis) (McConnel, et al., 2016), seizures, and acute esophageal injury (Bozzella, Magyar, DeBiasi, & Ferrer, 2020).

Formaldehyde, is classified as a carcinogen to humans by IARC and a probable human carcinogen by the EPA (ATSDR, 2020). Formaldehyde affects the gastrointestinal, immunological, and respiratory systems (ATSDR, 2020). Exposure to formaldehyde can irritate the skin, throat, lungs, and eyes, while repeated exposure to formaldehyde can lead to certain types of cancers (NIOSH, 2014). Benzene is also a classified carcinogen by the EPA and IARC (ATSDR, 2020). Health effects associated with exposure to benzene include effects on the hematological, immunological, and neurological systems. Exposure to benzene affects the eyes, skin, airway, nervous system, and lungs, and can result in blood cancers such as leukemia (Health,

2019). Acrolein is not a classifiable carcinogen by IARC or the EPA due to the lack of available evidence to assess potential carcinogenicity (ATSDR, 2020); however, health effects associated with exposure to acrolein include effects on the cardiovascular, hematological, ocular, and respiratory systems (ATSDR, 2020).

Toxic substances detected in e-cigarettes

Toxic substances detected in e-cigarettes include toxicants (chemicals, nanoparticles, and heavy metals) and toxins (endotoxin and β-glucans) [1]: Acetoin, Diacetyl, 2,3-Pentanedione (Allen et al., 2016); Glycerol, Formaldehyde and Acetaldehyde, Propylene glycerol (Klager et al., 2017); Nanoparticles, Carbonyls, volatile organic compounds – VOCs (Lee et al., 2017); endotoxins, β-glucans (Lee et al., 2019); heavy metals, polycyclic aromatic hydrocarbons – PAHs (Fowles et al., 2020); β-glucans (Lee and Christiani et al., 2020).

Nearly 300 compounds were identified in the aerosols of the 49 flavors, and the 10 compounds most highly correlated with radical production were selected for further investigation (Bitzer, et al., 2018).

Carbonyl compounds were found in the aerosol. These compounds have been implicated in the development of oxidative stress and release of inflammatory mediators,[2,3] increasing cardiovascular risk[4, 5, 6] and platelet function alteration,[7] airway epithelial injury, and creating disturbances in gas exchange function.[8]

Diacetyl and its structural analogs (2,3-pentadione, 2,3-hexanedione, and 2,3-heptanedione) are commonly used in buttery or caramellic flavored e-liquids (Ind, 2020). Diacetyl is associated with the severe respiratory disease bronchiolitis obliterans observed in popcorn factory workers (Barrington-Trimis, Samet, & McConnell, 2014; Fowles & DiBartolomeis, 2017). Additionally, research by Potera (2012) suggests that diacetyl substitutes may be just as toxic to the lung as diacetyl. Diacetyl substitutes have also been associated with adverse respiratory outcomes (Stratton, et al., 2018). Another study by Farsalinos, Kistler, Gillman, and Voudris (2015) concluded that daily inhaled exposures of diacetyl and 2,3-pentadione in e-liquids exceeded NIOSH recommended standards.

E-liquids come in many different flavors. Evaluation of nine different studies that investigated the chemical composition of over 670 flavored e-liquids identified ethyl maltol, ethyl vanillin, vanillin, cinnamaldehyde, and menthol as the most common flavoring chemicals (Aszyk, et al., 2018; Behar, Luo, McWhirter, Pankow, & Talbot, 2018; Bitzer, et al., 2018; Czoli, et al., 2019; Hua, et al., 2019; Hutzler, et al., 2014; Lisko, Tran, Stanfill, Blount, & Watson, 2015; Omaiye, et al., 2019; Tierney, Karpinski, Brown, Luo, & Pankow, 2016). In these nine studies, there were between 1 and 47 different flavoring chemicals detected in a single e-liquid. Comparison of flavor chemical concentrations of 476 e-liquids from seven individual studies identified concentrations from < 5 to 1.55 x 105 ppm (Aszyk, et al., 2018; Behar, et al., 2018; Bitzer, et al., 2018; Hua, et al., 2019; Lisko, et al., 2015; Omaiye, et al., 2019; Tierney, et al., 2016). Cinnamaldehyde, menthol, ethyl maltol, benzyl alcohol, and vanillin had the highest average reported concentrations which typically exceeded reported concentrations found in food or consumer products (Good-Scents-Company, 2021).

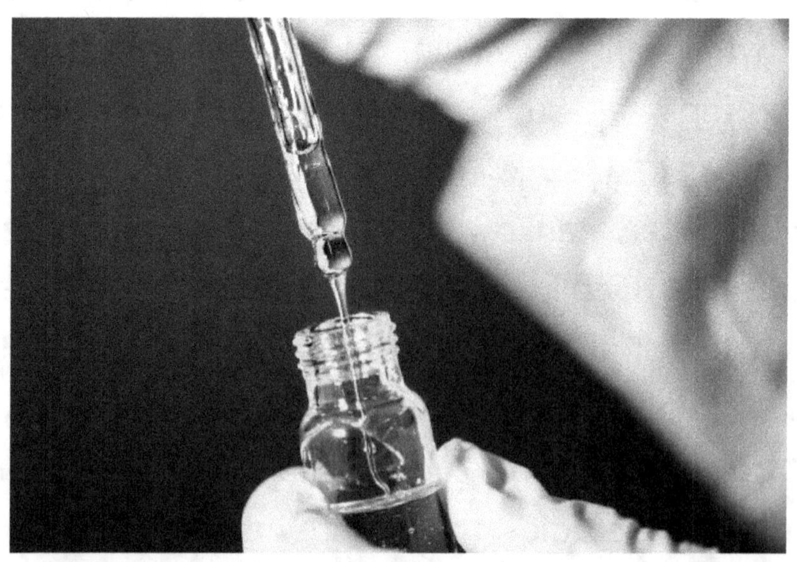

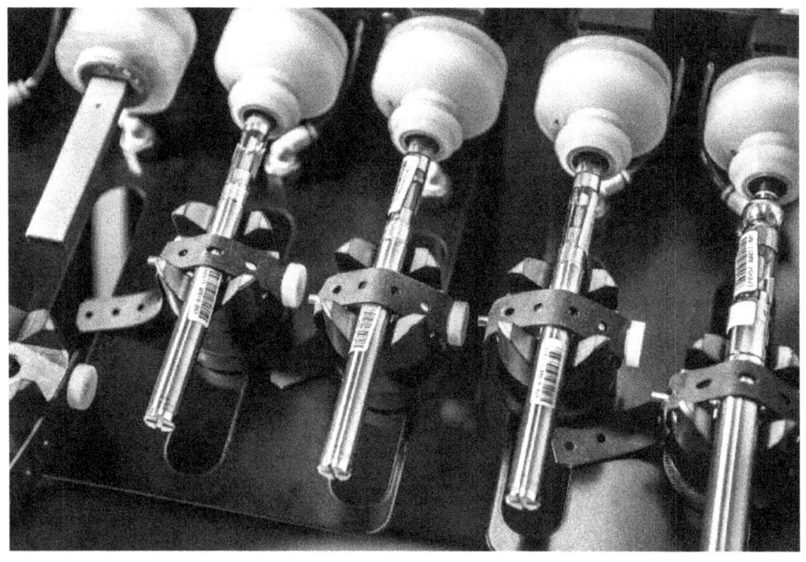

and vaping pens, that were undergoing tests inside a Centers for Disease Control and Prevention (CDC) laboratory.

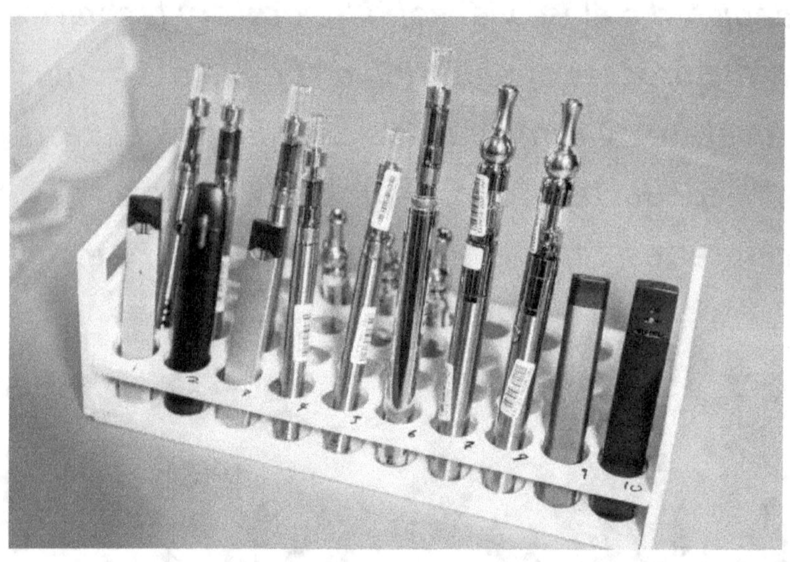

Public Health Image Library (PHIL), 23262 This image depicted a test tube rack that had been stocked with examples of various electronic cigarettes, referred to as e-cigarettes, or e-cigs, and vaping pens. These items would undergo testing inside a Centers for Disease Control and Prevention (CDC) laboratory environment.

The presence of metals and metalloids (e.g., arsenic, chromium, lead, nickel) in ENDS aerosols is a major concern, given their serious health effects, including cancer (Garcia-Esquinas, et al., 2014; Kuo, Moon, Wang, Silbergeld, & Navas-Acien, 2017), cardiovascular disease (Chowdhury, et al., 2018; Moon, Guallar, & Navas-Acien, 2012), renal damage (Suwazono, et al., 2006), and neurotoxicity (Caito & Aschner, 2015).

Almost any combination of chemicals can be found in the e-liquids that are currently on the market, since hundreds of chemicals are added to generate flavors that appeal to every man, woman, and kid from every nation and culture on Earth. While some chemical additions have never been given the go-ahead to be consumed by humans, others have been cleared for ingestion through the digestive system. The gastrointestinal tract has developed to prevent the body from absorbing poisons and being injured by them entering the body in this way, thus approval for gastrointestinal ingestion does not convey safety for inhaling the substances. [1]

However, adding chemicals to e-liquids for aerosolization and inhalation into the airways is taking advantage of this evolutionary process to quickly deliver the chemicals in e-cigarette aerosols into the bloodstream.[12] This is because the lungs have evolved to allow passage of molecules entering the airways directly into the bloodstream. [1]

Puff topography, which influences coil temperature and hence the makeup of e-cigarette emissions, is another factor associated with vaping exposure. While vaping e-cigarettes involves a longer inhalation (2.3–4.3 s), with many different intervals between puffs, the topography of smoking conventional tobacco cigarettes is similar among users: rapid (1–1.5 s) puffs, spaced by intervals of 20–30 s until the cigarette is finished, followed by either another cigarette or a break in between cigarettes.[13-

15] Although some e-cigarette users (vapers) are social vapers, only using e-cigarettes around friends or at parties, others vape continuously, with the first use before getting out of bed and the last use before bedtime. In addition, some people are exposed to secondhand e-cigarette aerosols, such that they are primarily inhaling aerosols that have entered someone else's lungs first. With the lack of sidestream vapor, because e-cigarettes only generate aerosols while the user is actively applying negative pressure to the mouthpiece, secondhand exposure to e-cigarette aerosols is likely to be less intense than that seen with cigarette smoke (which includes both sidestream and exhaled residual smoke). However, studies to date have confirmed that individuals standing close to e-cigarette users or within a confined space (a car or room without good ventilation) undergo significant exposure to e-cigarette aerosols. [16-18]

Interestingly, many e-cigarette users are not committed to a single device or a single flavor. Thus, they expose themselves to chemicals produced by multiple e-devices, plus the multitude of chemicals within the flavored e-liquids they choose to use. This complexity of e-cigarette use makes it more challenging to track sources of lung injury and inflammation caused by any single device or chemical. Finally, many e-cigarette users are also conventional tobacco smokers, marijuana smokers, or vapers of THC. Each of these inhalants has its own range of host effects, known and unknown, and the consequences of combining the various inhalants are yet unknown. [1]

Epidemiology of ALI from Vaping

Global usage of ENDS has increased in the last decade, especially among youth and young adults. [48] In 2019, the prevalence of ENDS among middle and high school studentsin the United States was 10.5 and 27.5%, respectively.[49] ENDS are noncombustible tobacco products that heat and aerosolize a liquid containing humectants and solvents. [26-28, 50]

In 2019, there were several outbreaks of acute respiratory failure of mysterious cause in persons who vape THC, nicotine, or both. Layden et al. [19] reported in the New England Journal of Medicine a cluster of cases from Illinois and Wisconsin in which patients presented with acute, severe respiratory distress after using e-cigarette products. Simultaneously released letters provided additional proof of this novel respiratory ailment caused by vaping: one reported six-case cluster from Utah [20] and the other detailed imaging alterations observed in a variety of instances. [21] Since then, the US Centers for Disease Control and Prevention (CDC) have dubbed the syndrome EVALI. A total of 2,602 hospitalized EVALI cases were recorded by the CDC as of January 9, 2020, in all 50 states, the District of Columbia (DC), and two territories (Puerto Rico and US Virgin Islands). By then, 27 states and Washington, DC have verified fifty-seven deaths. [1]

CDC Case Definitions for EVALI Surveillance

<u>Confirmed Case</u>

• E-cigarette/vaping use within 90 d of symptom onset,

• Radiograph opacities, pulmonary infiltrates in the chest or ground-glass opacities on chest CT,

• No evidence of other pulmonary infections,

• Patient medical history does not indicate an alternative diagnosis.

<u>Probable Case</u>

• E-cigarette/vaping use within 90 d of symptom onset,

• Radiograph opacities, pulmonary infiltrates in the chest or ground-glass opacities on chest CT,

• Evidence of infection, but the clinical team deems the infection is not likely the cause of the respiratory symptoms, or if testing for infectious agents were not performed,

• Patient medical history does not indicate an alternative diagnosis. (CDC)

Clinical presentation of EVALI

The primary symptoms of EVALI in patients are dyspnea, coughing, chest discomfort, diarrhea, abdominal pain, fever, and exhaustion [64, 65]. The onset of symptoms might happen hours or weeks before a presentation. Elevated erythrocyte sedimentation rate, c-reactive protein level, transaminitis, and leukocytosis are frequently found in laboratory testing [64]. Patients must have vaped within 90 days prior to the onset of symptoms, show bilateral infiltrates on chest imaging, have an infection evaluation that is negative, and have no other likely diagnosis in order to meet the CDC criteria for a "confirmed" EVALI case.

Coronal enhanced CT images through the anterior and posterior lungs show multifocal ground-glass opacity in the bilateral anterior upper lobes; conspicuous subpleural sparing. The posterior lungs show more pronounced consolidation with developing organization, evidenced by the mild architectural distortion and the band-like nature of the consolidation distributed along the bronchi. Coronal maximum intensity projected unenhanced computed tomography in a different EVALI patient shows diffusely distributed, small, centrilobular ground-glass opacity nodules typical of a non-fibrotic hypersensitivity pneumonitis pattern. [66]

BAL specimens from EVALI patients are mostly inflammatory with the majority of inflammatory cells being macrophages. Rare neutrophils, lymphocytes, and eosinophils may be encountered. The macrophages are unique in that their cytoplasm is often distended with mostly fine cytoplasmic vacuoles of similar size [67]. Enlarged cytoplasmic vacuoles and variably sized vacuoles, features seen in exogenous lipoid pneumonia, are encountered much less frequently. Oil red-O staining highlights the vacuoles to be composed of lipid material. The lipid-laden macrophage that was first feature associated with E-cigarette use in 2012 based only on clinical presentation, imaging findings, presence of lipid-laden macrophages, and a history of E-cigarette use [68].

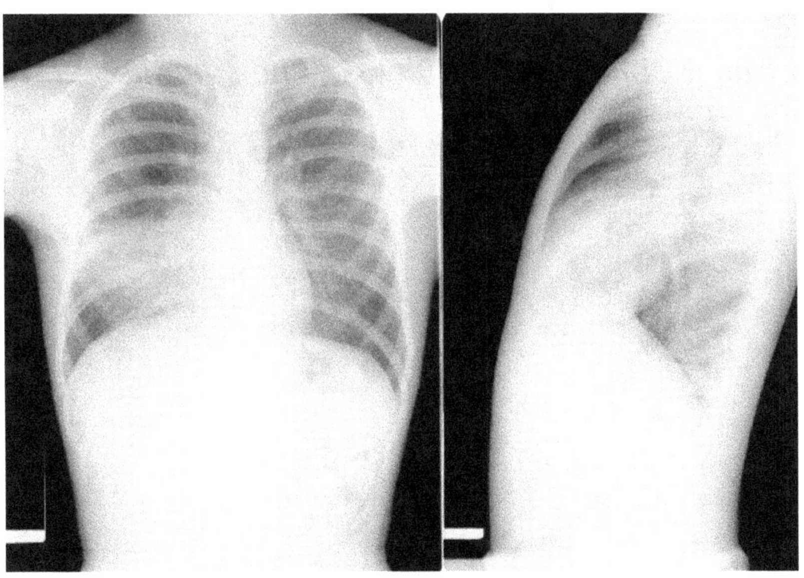

Public Health Image Library (PHIL), 21525. Not EVALI. This image depicted two chest x-rays, which revealed pathologic changes in a patient's

lung fields due to a condition known as mycoplasma pneumonia, caused by a Mycoplasma pneumoniae bacterial infection. Note on the anteroposterior (AP) view on the left, the generalized infiltrate permeating both lung fields, and consolidation in the region of the right lower lobe, as well as bilateral hilar adenopathy. In the left lateral view on the right, you can see that the consolidation occupied more of the posterior aspect of the lung fields, almost obliterating a view of the spinal column.

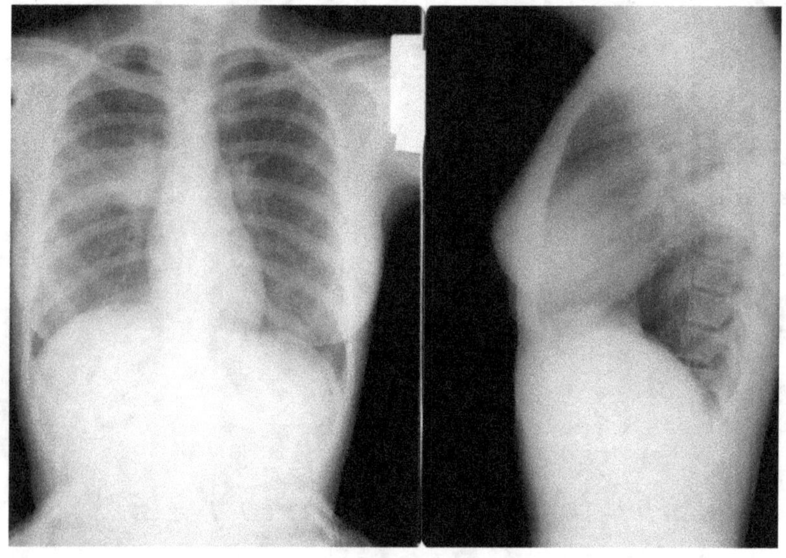

Public Health Image Library (PHIL), 21523. Not EVALI. This image depicted both an

In very early stages of acute lung injury, the only visible histologic finding may be edema and slightly enlarged pneumocytes. This is followed by the formation of hyaline membranes and fibrin deposition in the exudative phase. The proliferative, or organizing, phase shows the infiltration of inflammatory cells into the injurious process with subsequent polyps of organizing immature fibroblastic tissue. From a pathologic perspective, EVALI cases may show features of any of the patterns of acute lung injury, including diffuse alveolar damage, acute fibrinous and organizing pneumonia (AFOP), and organizing pneumonia. Some cases show distinctly airway-centered pathology, while others appear as more of a diffuse process. The relative presence of exudative and organizing features, along with the distribution of injury likely depends on (a) the temporal relationship between the toxic exposure (or repetitive toxic exposure) and the biopsy and (b) the severity/dose of the exposure. Cases of diffuse alveolar damage in the organizing phase may mimic cellular non-specific interstitial pneumonia.

Pathologic acute lung injury patterns seen in the setting of electronic cigarette or vaping-associated lung injury: https://www.ncbi.nlm.nih.gov/pmc/articles/PMC7590536/#CR19

The findings of high-resolution computed tomography are often ground-glass opacities and interlobular septal thickening reflecting emulating crazy paving, although pulmonary nodules have been reported. (Flower, M. et al., 2020)

Respiratory bronchiolitis-associated interstitial lung disease secondary to electronic nicotine delivery system use confirmed with open lung biopsy.[69]

Laboratory findings include leukocytosis; however, acute phase reactants and other markers of inflammation are not frequently requested. [10]

Treatment of EVALI

The best treatment is unknown because, due to the novelty of EVALI, treatment has only been examined in observational studies and case series. Extracorporeal membrane oxygenation (ECMO) was rarely necessary in a large group of 98 EVALI patients, with 76% requiring supplemental oxygen, 22% requiring noninvasive ventilation, and 26% requiring intubation and mechanical ventilation [70]. Most EVALI patients had a history of using systemic glucocorticoids [70, 71]. Despite the fact that there have been over sixty recorded deaths from EVALI, many individuals may get symptom relief when they stop vaping [72].

Usually, coverage of broad-spectrum antibiotics is provided, suggesting a concomitant infectious process. [10]

Coverage with broad-spectrum antibiotics is encouraged with sequential de-escalation if no evidence of respiratory tract or systemic infection is found. It is imperative to monitor ventilator-induced lung injury, especially when clinical deterioration justifies more aggressive measurements. Overdistension of the alveoli from either high positive end-expiratory pressure (PEEP) or high tidal volumes can lead to volutrauma, and simultaneously an excessive airway pressure can result in pneumothorax. Likewise, oxygen should be titrated to a minimal arterial oxygen tension of 65 mm Hg to reduce the risk of oxygen toxicity. [10]

Assessment of the pulmonary mechanics needs to be mandatory. Important tools such as driving pressure, esophageal balloon, and stress index can give us critical information on the patient's needs. The management should be personalized and tailored to each patient's physiology. The prone position needs to be implemented when indicated with no delay as well as neuromuscular blockade. Fluid restriction and adequate nutrition are crucial. Furthermore, health care providers have to be attentive to superimposed complications such as ventilator-associated pneumonia. Extracorporeal membrane oxygenation may be necessary depending on the severity of illness. [73, 74] Finally, a multidisciplinary approach is vital to improve chances of intensive care unit survival. Implementing strategies such as ABCDEF bundle [75] and coordinating multidisciplinary care should be the cornerstone of management. [10]

According to some data, the care that the patients with EVALI required during hospitalization included supplemental oxygen, a high-flow nasal cannula, noninvasive positive pressure ventilation, intubation and mechanical ventilation, intensive care unit care, initiation of antibiotics, and steroids.[84]

The CDC and the Lung Injury Response Clinical Working group have established an algorithm for the management of patients with EVALI to improve outcomes, reduce hospital readmission, and prevent death (https://www.cdc.gov/tobacco/basic_informatio n/e-cigarettes/pdfs/Algorithm-EVALI-Dec-2019-p.pdf). The guidance includes diagnosis, inpatient and outpatient management, postdischarge follow-up and support, and considerations for seasonal influenza. The CDC offers suggestions on questions to ask during the initial clinical assessment to obtain information essential for an EVALI diagnosis (https://www.cdc.gov/tobacco/basic_informatio

n/e-cigarettes/severe-lung-disease/healthcare-providers/pdfs/dont-forget-to-ask-assessing-the-risk-of-lung-injury-508.pdf).

Prognosis and long-term consequences

Studies investigating imaging abnormalities in ARDS survivors have shown that the disease can resolve completely. The degree of resolution reported among different studies varies widely, with between 25 and 85% of ARDS survivors reported to have residual fibrotic changes on chest imaging [76, 77]. Therefore, it is hypothesized that a fraction of EVALI survivors may develop similar chronic fibrotic changes, but long-term studies will be needed to investigate this hypothesis. Clinical and imaging follow-up will be critical to ensure resolution of the pathologic process. Case reports have suggested that there may be residual lung dysfunction, mainly diffusion abnormalities, present for at least up to 2 months after discharge [78, 79].

According to some data, the median age of the patients who died was higher than those who were readmitted to the hospital or were neither readmitted nor died. [83] The patients who died or were readmitted to the hospital had a history of one or more chronic conditions. [83] These conditions included cardiac disease, obstructive sleep apnea, and chronic obstructive pulmonary disease for patients who died. [82]

Prevention of lung injuries

During hospitalization, patients should abstain from e-cigarette and vaping products and antimicrobial agents and corticosteroids should be initiated as the condition warrants. [82]

Patients should also be offered an influenza vaccination, if applicable. These include pharmacists to ensure medications are being taken as prescribed (i.e., corticosteroids) and outpatient follow-up appointments within 48 hours of discharge with a primary care physician and at 2 to 4 weeks with a pulmonologist. Patients should be urged not to use e-cigarettes or vaping products, as these could cause a recurrence of respiratory symptoms, with substance abuse support and clinically proven methods of smoking cessation. Considerations for outpatient care include chest radiograph, influenza virus testing, stopping e-cigarette and/or vaping use, corticosteroids, smoking cessation support, influenza vaccination, and 24 to 48 hours follow-up with a primary care physician. [82]

All persons, including patients with cancer, should quit smoking by using a clinically proven cessation strategy, that is, pharmacotherapy or counseling. Constituents of e-cigarette liquids may contribute to adverse health effects associated with vaping, and e-cigarettes should not be used by adolescents or adults who do not currently smoke.

Conclusion

The use of illicit drugs, addiction, and the start of tobacco usage among nonsmokers are all possible consequences of using electronic cigarette devices. Different electronic cigarette ingredients can have negative consequences that extend beyond the respiratory system. [10]

EVALI is a serious respiratory illness that, in its most severe form, manifests as acute respiratory distress syndrome [80]. As of right now, there is mounting proof that e-cigarettes harm and inflame the lungs in addition to having negative systemic effects on several organs. Prior to EVALI, vaping had been associated with a wide variety of pulmonary presentations including lipoid pneumonia, acute respiratory distress syndrome, and diffuse alveolar hemorrhage. However, the majority of the cases of EVALI are likely related to vaping VEA.

The EVALI outbreak highlights the importance of regulation of these products by agencies, including the United States Food and Drug Administration, and the importance of these regulations and efforts to reduce use of these products through taxation, education, and other efforts. [82]

There is clear scientific evidence that these devices pose a risk to the physical and mental health of children and adolescents. [105]

E-cigarette use can be profoundly hazardous. Exposure to EC aerosol can be fatally harmful.

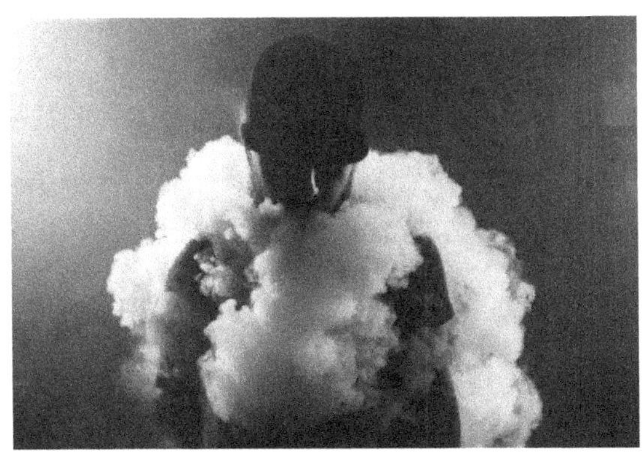

References

1. Park JA, Crotty Alexander LE, Christiani DC. Vaping and Lung Inflammation and Injury. Annu Rev Physiol. 2022 Feb 10;84:611-629. doi: 10.1146/annurev-physiol-061121-040014. Epub 2021 Nov 1. PMID: 34724436; PMCID: PMC10228557.

2. Singh, S. Brocker, C. Koppaka, V.... Aldehyde dehydrogenases in cellular responses to oxidative/electrophilic stress. Free Radic Biol Med. 2013; 56:89-101.

3. Carnevale, R. Sciarretta, S. Violi, F. ... Acute impact of tobacco vs electronic cigarette smoking on oxidative stress and vascular function. Chest. 2016; 150:606-612.

4. Olfert, I.M. DeVallance, E. Hoskinson, H. ... Chronic exposure to electronic cigarettes results in impaired cardiovascular function in mice. J Appl Physiol (1985). 2018; 124:573-582.

5. Bhatta, D.N. Glantz, S.A. Electronic cigarette use and myocardial infarction among adults in the us population assessment of tobacco and health. J Am Heart Assoc. 2019; 8:e012317.

6. MacDonald, A. Middlekauff, H.R. Electronic cigarettes and cardiovascular health: what do we know so far? Vasc Health Risk Manag. 2019; 15:159-174.

7. Hom, S. Chen, L. Wang, T. ... Platelet activation, adhesion, inflammation, and aggregation potential are altered in the presence of electronic cigarette extracts of variable nicotine concentrations. Platelets. 2016; 27:694-702.

8. Chaumont, M. van de Borne, P. Bernard, A. ... Fourth generation e-cigarette vaping induces transient lung inflammation and gas exchange disturbances: results from two randomized clinical trials. Am J Physiol Lung Cell Mol Physiol. 2019; 316:L705-L719.

9. Bonner E, Chang Y, Christie E, Colvin V, Cunningham B, Elson D, Ghetu C, Huizenga J, Hutton SJ, Kolluri SK, Maggio S, Moran I, Parker B, Rericha Y, Rivera BN, Samon S, Schwichtenberg T, Shankar P, Simonich MT, Wilson LB, Tanguay RL. The chemistry and toxicology of vaping. Pharmacol Ther. 2021 Sep;225:107837. doi: 10.1016/j.pharmthera.2021.107837. Epub 2021 Mar 19. PMID: 33753133; PMCID: PMC8263470.

10. Fonseca Fuentes X, Kashyap R, Hays JT, Chalmers S, Lama von Buchwald C, Gajic O, Gallo de Moraes A. VpALI-Vaping-related Acute Lung Injury: A New Killer Around the Block. Mayo Clin Proc. 2019 Dec;94(12):2534-2545. doi: 10.1016/j.mayocp.2019.10.010. Epub 2019 Nov 22. PMID: 31767123.

11. Dockrell M, Morrison R, Bauld L, McNeill A. 2013. E-cigarettes: prevalence and attitudes in GreatBritain. Nicotine Tob. Res 15:1737–44.

12. Grana R, Benowitz N, Glantz SA. 2014. E-cigarettes: a scientific review. Circulation 129:1972–86.

13. Zhu SH, Sun JY, Bonnevie E, Cummins SE, Gamst A, et al. 2014. Four hundred and sixty brands ofe-cigarettes and counting: implications for product regulation. Tob. Control 23(Suppl. 3):iii3–9.

14. Hajek P, Etter JF, Benowitz N, Eissenberg T, McRobbie H. 2014. Electronic cigarettes: review of use,content, safety, effects on smokers and potential for harm and benefit. Addiction 109:1801–10.

15. Shahandeh N, Chowdhary H, Middlekauff HR. 2021. Vaping and cardiac disease. Heart 107:1530–35.

16. Choi H, Lin Y, Race E, Macmurdo MG. 2021. Electronic cigarettes and alternative methods of vaping. Ann. Am. Thorac. Soc 18:191–99.

17. DeVito EE, Krishnan-Sarin S. 2018. E-cigarettes: impact of e-liquid components and device characteristics on nicotine exposure. Curr. Neuropharmacol 16:438–59.

18. Vreeke S, Zhu X, Strongin RM. 2020. A simple predictive model for estimating relative e-cigarette toxic carbonyl levels. PLOS ONE 15:e0238172.

19. Zhao D, Aravindakshan A, Hilpert M, Olmedo P, Rule AM, et al. 2020. Metal/metalloid levels in electronic cigarette liquids, aerosols, and human biosamples: a systematic review. Environ. Health Perspect 128:36001.

20. Olmedo P, Goessler W, Tanda S, Grau-Perez M, Jarmul S, et al. 2018. Metal concentrations in e-cigarette liquid and aerosol samples: the contribution of metallic coils. Environ. Health Perspect 126:027010.

21. Lerner CA, Sundar IK, Watson RM, Elder A, Jones R, et al. 2015. Environmental health hazards of e-cigarettes and their components:

oxidants and copper in e-cigarette aerosols. Environ. Pollut 198:100–7.

22. Fowles J, Barreau T, Wu N. 2020. Cancer and non-cancer risk concerns from metals in electronic cigarette liquids and aerosols. Int. J. Environ. Res. Public Health 17:2146.

23. Allen JG, Flanigan SS, LeBlanc M, Vallarino J, MacNaughton P, et al. 2016. Flavoring chemicals in e-cigarettes: diacetyl, 2,3-pentanedione, and acetoin in a sample of 51 products, including fruit-, candy-, and cocktail-flavored e-cigarettes. Environ. Health Perspect 124:733–39.

24. Klager S, Vallarino J, MacNaughton P, Christiani DC, Lu Q, Allen JG 2017. Flavoring chemicals and aldehydes in e-cigarette emissions. Environ. Sci. Technol 51:10806–13.

25. Lee MS, LeBouf RF, Son YS, Koutrakis P, Christiani DC. 2017. Nicotine, aerosol particles, carbonyls and volatile organic compounds in tobacco- and menthol-flavored e-cigarettes. Environ. Health 16:42.

26. Lee MS,Allen JG,Christiani DC.2019.Endotoxin and (1 → 3)-β-d-glucan contamination in electronic cigarette products sold in the United States. Environ. Health Perspect 127:47008.

27. Lee MS, Christiani DC. 2020. Microbial toxins in nicotine vaping liquids. Am. J. Respir. Crit. Care Med 201:741–43.

28. Kennedy CD,van Schalkwyk MCI,McKee M,Pisinger C.2019.The cardiovascular effects of electronic cigarettes: a systematic review of experimental studies. Prev. Med 127:105770.

29. Bergeria CL, Heil SH, Bunn JY, Sigmon SC, Higgins ST. 2018. Comparing smoking topography and subjective measures of usual brand cigarettes between pregnant and non-pregnant smokers.Nicotine Tob. Res 20:1243–49.

30. Cox S, Goniewicz ML, Kosmider L, McRobbie H, Kimber C, Dawkins L. 2021. The time course of compensatory puffing with an electronic

cigarette: secondary analysis of real-world puffing data with highandlownicotineconcentrationunderfixedand adjustablepowersettings.NicotineTob.Res 23:1153–59.

31. Glasser AM, Johnson AL, Niaura RS, Abrams DB, Pearson JL. 2021. Youth vaping and tobacco use in context in the United States: results from the 2018 National Youth Tobacco Survey. Nicotine Tob. Res 23:447–53.

32. Ballbe M, Martinez-Sanchez JM, Sureda X, Fu M, Perez-Ortuno R, et al. 2014. Cigarettes versus e-cigarettes: passive exposure at home measured by means of airborne marker and biomarkers. Environ. Res 135:76–80.

33. Lee MS, Rees VW, Koutrakis P, Wolfson JM, Son YS, et al. 2019. Cardiac autonomic effects of second-hand exposure to nicotine from electronic cigarettes: an exploratory study. Environ. Epidemiol 3:e033.

34. Visser WF, Klerx WN, Cremers H, Ramlal R, Schwillens PL, Talhout R. 2019. The health risks of electronic cigarette use to bystanders. Int. J. Environ. Res. Public Health 16:1525.

35. Layden JE, Ghinai I, Pray I, Kimball A, Layer M, et al. 2020. Pulmonary illness related to e-cigarette use in Illinois and Wisconsin—Final Report. N. Engl. J. Med 382:903–16.

36. Maddock SD, Cirulis MM, Callahan SJ, Keenan LM, Pirozzi CS, et al. 2019. Pulmonary lipid-laden macrophages and vaping. N. Engl. J. Med 381:1488–89.

37. Henry TS, Kanne JP, Kligerman SJ. 2019. Imaging of vaping-associated lung disease. N. Engl. J. Med 381:1486–87.

38. Mull ES, Erdem G, Nicol K, Adler B, Shell R. 2020. Eosinophilic pneumonia and lymphadenopathy associated with vaping and tetrahydrocannabinol use. Pediatrics 145:e20193007.

39. Collins BN, Lepore SJ, Winickoff JP, Nair US, Moughan B, et al. 2018. An office-initiated multilevel intervention for tobacco smoke exposure: a randomized trial. Pediatrics 141:S75–86.

40. Galiatsatos P, Gomez E, Lin CT, Illei PB, Shah P, Neptune E. 2020. Secondhand smoke from electronic cigarette resulting in hypersensitivity pneumonitis. BMJ Case Rep. 13:e233381.

41. Christiani DC. 2020. Vaping-induced acute lung injury. N. Engl. J. Med 382:960–62.

42. De Giacomi F, Vassallo R, Yi ES, Ryu JH. 2018. Acute eosinophilic pneumonia. Causes, diagnosis, and management. Am. J. Respir. Crit. Care Med 197:728–36.

43. Blount BC, Karwowski MP, Shields PG, Morel-Espinosa M, Valentin-Blasini L, et al. 2020. Vitamin E acetate in bronchoalveolar-lavage fluid associated with EVALI. N. Engl. J. Med 382:697–705.

44. Bhat TA, Kalathil SG, Bogner PN, Blount BC, Goniewicz ML, Thanavala YM. 2020. An animal model of inhaled vitamin E acetate and EVALI-like lung injury. N. Engl. J. Med 382:1175–77.

45. Reagan-Steiner S, Gary J, Matkovic E, Ritter JM, Shieh WJ, et al. 2020. Pathological findings in suspected cases of e-cigarette, or vaping, product use-associated lung injury (EVALI): a case series. Lancet Respir. Med 8:1219–32.

46. Mukhopadhyay S, Mehrad M, Dammert P, Arrossi AV, Sarda R, et al. 2020. Lung biopsy findings in severe pulmonary illness associated with e-cigarette use (vaping). Am. J. Clin. Pathol 153:30–39.

47. Gaiha SM, Cheng J, Halpern-Felsher B. 2020. Association between youth smoking, electronic cigarette use, and COVID-19. J. Adolesc. Health 67:519–23.

48. Besaratinia A, Tommasi S. 2019. Vaping: a growing global health concern. E Clinical Medicine 17:100208.

49. Cullen KA, Gentzke AS, Sawdey MD, Chang JT, Anic GM, et al. 2019. E-cigarette use among youth in the United States, 2019. JAMA 322:2095–103.

50. Hwang JH, Lyes M, Sladewski K, Enany S, McEachern E, et al. 2016. Electronic cigarette inhalation alters innate immunity and airway cytokines while increasing the virulence of colonizing bacteria. J. Mol. Med 94:667–79.

51. Park HR, O'Sullivan M, Vallarino J, Shumyatcher M, Himes BE, et al. 2019. Transcriptomic response of primary human airway epithelial cells to flavoring chemicals in electronic cigarettes. Sci. Rep 9:1400.

52. Schweitzer RJ, Wills TA, Tam E, Pagano I, Choi K. 2017. E-cigarette use and asthma in a multi-ethnic sample of adolescents. Prev. Med 105:226–31.

53. Osei AD, Mirbolouk M, Orimoloye OA, Dzaye O, Uddin SMI, et al. 2019. The association between e-cigarette use and asthma among

never combustible cigarette smokers: behavioral risk factor surveillance system (BRFSS) 2016 & 2017. BMC Pulm. Med 19:180.

54. Cho JH, Paik SY. 2016. Association between electronic cigarette use and asthma among high school students in South Korea. PLOS ONE 11:e0151022.

55. Choi K, Bernat D. 2016. E-cigarette use among Florida youth with and without asthma. Am. J. Prev. Med 51:446–53.

56. Li D, Xie Z. 2020. Cross-sectional association of lifetime electronic cigarette use with wheezing and related respiratory symptoms in U.S. adults. Nicotine Tob. Res 22:S85–92.

57. Staudt MR, Salit J, Kaner RJ, Hollmann C, Crystal RG. 2018. Altered lung biology of healthy never smokers following acute inhalation of E-cigarettes. Respir. Res 19:78.

58. Larcombe AN. 2019. Early-life exposure to electronic cigarettes: cause for concern. Lancet Respir. Med 7:985–92.

59. Wetendorf M, Randall LT, Lemma MT, Hurr SH, Pawlak JB, et al. 2019. E-cigarette exposure delays implantation and causes reduced weight gain in female offspring exposed in utero.J.Endocr.Soc 3:1907–16.

60. McGrath-Morrow SA,Gorzkowski J,Groner JA,Rule AM,Wilson K,et al.2020.The effects of nicotine on development. Pediatrics 145:e20191346.

61. Meyer KF, Verkaik-Schakel RN, Timens W, Kobzik L, Plosch T, Hylkema MN. 2017. The fetal programming effect of prenatal smoking on Igf1r and Igf1 methylation is organ- and sex-specific. Epigenetics 12:1076–91.

62. Holbrook BD. 2016. The effects of nicotine on human fetal development. Birth Defects Res. C Embryo Today 108:181–92.

63. Wong MK, Barra NG, Alfaidy N, Hardy DB, Holloway AC. 2015. Adverse effects of perinatal nicotine exposure on reproductive outcomes. Reproduction 150:R185–93.

64. Crotty Alexander LE, et al., (2020) NIH workshop report: E-cigarette or vaping product use associated lung injury (EVALI): developing a research agenda. Am J Respir Crit Care Med.

65. Kligerman S, et al. Radiologic, pathologic, clinical, and physiologic findings of electronic cigarette or vaping product use-associated lung injury (EVALI): evolving knowledge and remaining questions. Radiology. 2020;294(3):491–505. doi: 10.1148/radiol.2020192585.

66. Smith ML, Gotway MB, Crotty Alexander LE, Hariri LP. Vaping-related lung injury. Virchows Arch. 2021 Jan;478(1):81-88. doi: 10.1007/s00428-020-02943-0. Epub 2020 Oct 27. PMID: 33106908; PMCID: PMC7590536.

67. Saqi A, et al. E-cigarette or vaping product use-associated lung injury: what is the role of cytologic assessment? Cancer Cytopathol. 2020;128(6):371–380. doi: 10.1002/cncy.22237.

68. McCauley L, Markin C, Hosmer D. An unexpected consequence of electronic cigarette use. Chest. 2012;141(4):1110–1113. doi: 10.1378/chest.11-1334.

69. [published correction appears in Respirol Case Rep. 2017]Respirol Case Rep. 2017; 5:e00230.

70. Layden JE, et al. Pulmonary illness related to E-cigarette use in Illinois and Wisconsin - final report. N Engl J Med. 2020;382(10):903–916. doi: 10.1056/NEJMoa1911614.

71. Davidson K, et al. Outbreak of electronic-cigarette-associated acute lipoid pneumonia - North Carolina, July-august 2019. MMWR Morb Mortal Wkly Rep. 2019;68(36):784–786. doi:10.15585/mmwr.mm6836e1.

72. Alexander LEC, Perez MF (2019) Identifying, tracking, and treating lung injury associated with e-cigarettes or vaping. Lancet.

73. Attis, M. King, J. Hardison, D. ... The journey to ECMO could start with a single vape: a case of severe hypersensitivity pneumonitis in a pediatric patient. ASAIO J. 2018; 64:14.

74. Aokage, T. Tsukahara, K. Fukuda, Y. ... Heat-not-burn cigarettes induce fulminant acute eosinophilic pneumonia requiring extracorporeal membrane oxygenation. Respir Med Case Rep. 2018; 26:87-90.

75. Marra, A. Ely, E.W. Pandharipande, P.P. ... The ABCDEF bundle in critical care. Crit Care Clin. 2017; 33:225-243.

76. Desai SR, et al. Acute respiratory distress syndrome: CT abnormalities at long-term follow-up. Radiology. 1999;210(1):29–35. doi: 10.1148/radiology.210.1.r99ja2629.

77. Sheard S, Rao P, Devaraj A. Imaging of acute respiratory distress syndrome. Respir Care. 2012;57(4):607–612. doi: 10.4187/respcare.01731.

78. Carroll BJ, et al. Impaired lung function following e-cigarette or vaping product use associated lung injury in the first cohort of hospitalized adolescents. Pediatr Pulmonol. 2020;55(7):1712–1718. doi: 10.1002/ppul.24787.

79. Corcoran A, Carl JC, Rezaee F. The importance of anti-vaping vigilance-EVALI in seven adolescent pediatric patients in Northeast Ohio. Pediatr Pulmonol. 2020;55(7):1719–1724. doi: 10.1002/ppul.24872.

80. Chatham-Stephens K, et al. Characteristics of hospitalized and nonhospitalized patients in a nationwide outbreak of E-cigarette, or vaping, product use-associated lung injury - United States, November 2019. MMWR Morb Mortal

Wkly Rep. 2019;68(46):1076–1080. doi: 10.15585/mmwr.mm6846e1.

81. Petrella F, Rizzo S, Masiero M, Marzorati C, Casiraghi M, Bertolaccini L, Mazzella A, Pravettoni G, Spaggiari L. Clinical impact of vaping on cardiopulmonary function and lung cancer development: an update. Eur J Cancer Prev. 2023 Nov 1;32(6):584-589. doi: 10.1097/CEJ.0000000000000797. Epub 2023 Mar 21. PMID: 36942844.

82. Rice SJ, Hyland V, Behera M, Ramalingam SS, Bunn P, Belani CP. Guidance on the Clinical Management of Electronic Cigarette or Vaping-Associated Lung Injury. J Thorac Oncol. 2020 Nov;15(11):1727-1737. doi: 10.1016/j.jtho.2020.08.012. Epub 2020 Aug 29. PMID: 32866653; PMCID: PMC7455516.

83. Mikosz C.A., Danielson M., Anderson K.N., et al. Characteristics of patients experiencing rehospitalization or death after hospital discharge in a nationwide outbreak of e-

cigarette, or vaping, product use-associated lung injury - United States, 2019. MMWR Morb Mortal Wkly Rep. 2020;68:1183–1188.

84. Heinzerling A., Armatas C., Karmarkar E., et al. Severe lung injury associated with use of e-cigarette, or vaping, products - California, 2019. JAMA Intern Med. 2020;180:1–9.

85. Esteban-Lopez M, Perry MD, Garbinski LD, Manevski M, Andre M, Ceyhan Y, Caobi A, Paul P, Lau LS, Ramelow J, Owens F, Souchak J, Ales E, El-Hage N. Health effects and known pathology associated with the use of E-cigarettes. Toxicol Rep. 2022 Jun 16;9:1357-1368. doi: 10.1016/j.toxrep.2022.06.006. PMID: 36561957; PMCID: PMC9764206.

86. Besaratinia A., Tommasi S. Vaping: a growing global health concern. EClinicalMedicine. 2019;17 doi: 10.1016/j.eclinm.2019.10.019.

87. Euromonitor International. Smokless tobacco and vapour products2020 (accessed 2 Feb 2021). Available from:

⟨https://www.euromonitor.com/smokeless-tobacco-and-vapour-products⟩.

88. Villarroel M.A., Cha A.E., Vahratian A. Electronic cigarette use among U.S. adults, 2018. NCHS Data Brief. 2020;(365):1–8.

89. Gentzke A.S., Creamer M., Cullen K.A., Ambrose B.K., Willis G., Jamal A., et al. Vital signs: tobacco product use among middle and high school students - United States, 2011-2018. MMWR Morb. Mortal. Wkly. Rep. 2019;68(6) doi: 10.15585/mmwr.mm6806e1.

90. Kim A.E., Arnold K.Y., Makarenko O. E-cigarette advertising expenditures in the U.S., 2011-2012. Am. J. Prev. Med. 2014;46(4):409–412. doi: 10.1016/j.amepre.2013.11.003.

91. Truth Initiative. Vaporized:youth and young adult exposure to e-cigarette marketing.2015 (accessed 2 Feb 2021). Available from: ⟨https://truthinitiative.org/sites/default/files/media/files/2019/03/Vaporized-Youth-Exposure-To-E-Cigarette-Marketing.pdf⟩.

92. Singh T., Marynak K., Arrazola R.A., Cox S., Rolle I.V., King B.A. Vital signs: exposure to electronic cigarette advertising among middle school and high school students - United States, 2014. MMWR Morb. Mortal. Wkly. Rep. 2016;64(52):1403–1408. doi: 10.15585/mmwr.mm6452a3.

93. Mantey D.S., Cooper M.R., Clendennen S.L., Pasch K.E., Perry C.L. E-cigarette marketing exposure is associated with e-cigarette use among US youth. J. Adolesc. Health. 2016;58(6):686–690. doi: 10.1016/j.jadohealth.2016.03.003.

94. Cullen K.A., Gentzke A.S., Sawdey M.D., Chang J.T., Anic G.M., Wang T.W., et al. e-cigarette use among youth in the United States, 2019. JAMA. 2019;322(21):2095–2103. doi: 10.1001/jama.2019.18387.

95. Miech R., Johnston L., O'Malley P.M., Bachman J.G., Patrick M.E. Trends in adolescent vaping, 2017-2019. N Engl J Med.

2019;381(15):1490–1491. doi: 10.1056/NEJMc1910739.

96. Canistro D., Vivarelli F., Cirillo S., Babot Marquillas C., Buschini A., Lazzaretti M., et al. E-cigarettes induce toxicological effects that can raise the cancer risk. Sci. Rep. 2017;7(1):2028. doi: 10.1038/s41598-017-02317-8.

97. Kaisar M.A., Villalba H., Prasad S., Liles T., Sifat A.E., Sajja R.K., et al. Offsetting the impact of smoking and e-cigarette vaping on the cerebrovascular system and stroke injury: is Metformin a viable countermeasure. Redox Biol. 2017;13:353–362. doi: 10.1016/j.redox.2017.06.006.

98. Hua M., Sadah S., Hristidis V., Talbot P. Health effects associated with electronic cigarette use: automated mining of online forums. J. Med. Internet Res. 2020;22(1) doi: 10.2196/15684.

99. Franzen K.F., Willig J., Cayo Talavera S., Meusel M., Sayk F., Reppel M., et al. E-cigarettes

and cigarettes worsen peripheral and central hemodynamics as well as arterial stiffness: a randomized, double-blinded pilot study. Vasc. Med. 2018;23(5):419–425. doi: 10.1177/1358863x18779694.

100. Kuntic M., Oelze M., Steven S., Kröller-Schön S., Stamm P., Kalinovic S., et al. Short-term e-cigarette vapour exposure causes vascular oxidative stress and dysfunction: evidence for a close connection to brain damage and a key role of the phagocytic NADPH oxidase (NOX-2) Eur. Heart J. 2019:2472–2483. doi: 10.1093/eurheartj/ehz772.

101. Yu V., Rahimy M., Korrapati A., Xuan Y., Zou A.E., Krishnan A.R., et al. Electronic cigarettes induce DNA strand breaks and cell death independently of nicotine in cell lines. Oral Oncol. 2016;52:58–65. doi: 10.1016/j.oraloncology.2015.10.018.

102. Lee H.W., Park S.H., Weng M.W., Wang H.T., Huang W.C., Lepor H., et al. E-cigarette

smoke damages DNA and reduces repair activity in mouse lung, heart, and bladder as well as in human lung and bladder cells. Proc. Natl. Acad. Sci. USA. 2018;115(7):E1560–e9. doi: 10.1073/pnas.1718185115.

103. Schaal C.M., Bora-Singhal N., Kumar D.M., Chellappan S.P. Regulation of Sox2 and stemness by nicotine and electronic-cigarettes in non-small cell lung cancer. Mol. Cancer. 2018;17(1):149. doi: 10.1186/s12943-018-0901-2.

104. Banks E, Yazidjoglou A, Brown S, Nguyen M, Martin M, Beckwith K, Daluwatta A, Campbell S, Joshy G. Electronic cigarettes and health outcomes: umbrella and systematic review of the global evidence. Med J Aust. 2023 Apr 3;218(6):267-275. doi: 10.5694/mja2.51890. Epub 2023 Mar 20. PMID: 36939271; PMCID: PMC10952413.

105. Chong-Silva DC, Sant'Anna MFBP, Riedi CA, Sant'Anna CC, Ribeiro JD, Vieira LMN, Pinto LA,

Terse-Ramos R, Morgan MAP, Godinho RN, di Francesco RC, da Silva CAM, Urrutia-Pereira M, Lotufo JPB, Silva LR, Solé D. Electronic cigarettes: "wolves in sheep's clothing". J Pediatr (Rio J). 2024 Sep 5:S0021-7557(24)00106-2. doi: 10.1016/j.jped.2024.06.015. Epub ahead of print. PMID: 39245237.